Made in United States
Troutdale, OR
04/16/2024

19232412R00056